Twenty Classic Recipes "Gluten Free"
and
Gluten Free Product Reference Guide

L. Honeywell

Copyright

Acknowledgements

Many thanks to all the creative guides along the way who helped in transforming a bunch of ideas into a dream come true. Your infusion of excellence, expertise and love has taken a concept and created a valuable tool for many.

To Amanda Walden of Wordsworth Typing and Transcribing, thank you for your editing and typing.

To Mary Murphy, whose belief in me and ability to help people, along with invaluable encouragement and great ideas have empowered me to complete this book. Thank you, Mary.

To Dr. Kent Holtorf, whose expertise and discernment got to the "root" of my health problems, which inspired me to try a gluten free diet. Thank you for your belief in me and your never-ending compassion.

To my parents, Betty and Russ, the "taste testers" and critics of my recipes. Your patience and love and endurance is an inspiration to our family and all who know you. Mom, no one compares to you in the kitchen!

Introduction

Did I ever dream that I would be writing this simple little cookbook? Frankly, no. It never crossed my mind. When I was young, my mother taught me how to cook and to maintain a healthy diet. She was a great cook and my sisters and I never lacked any good thing when it came to food and a complete dinner on the table every day until I went away to college. At that point, I began to appreciate all the love and effort she put into her meals. So did my taste buds.

Getting creative in the kitchen happened after major digestive problems with no explanations for how my overall health was affected from undiagnosed food allergies. That is when I learned about food sensitivities. Not everyone suffers from these things, but to those who prefer to eat gluten free, I write this for them. Everyone deserves to enjoy eating and walking away from the table knowing that what they just did was for not only the benefit of their health but also for their enjoyment. In this short compilation of recipes I hope to bring back those easy to prepare classics for those who choose to eat gluten free. I also hope to make it very easy for those just starting out on a gluten free diet to have resources at their fingertips so they can embark on their new culinary journey stress free. To prepare a pleasurable meal is an art. To prepare a gluten free meal is a skill. I hope this provides all its readers with both.

Bon Appétit!

Table of Contents

Baked Breaded Sole Almondine

Ingredients:

6 sole fillets
2 1/2 C Crispy Chicken Mix (Gluten Free) by Kinnikinnick or Gluten Free Corn Breading
4 oz sliced almonds
2 eggs
1 C fat free milk
6 Tbsp Olivio Spread
(or butter substitute)

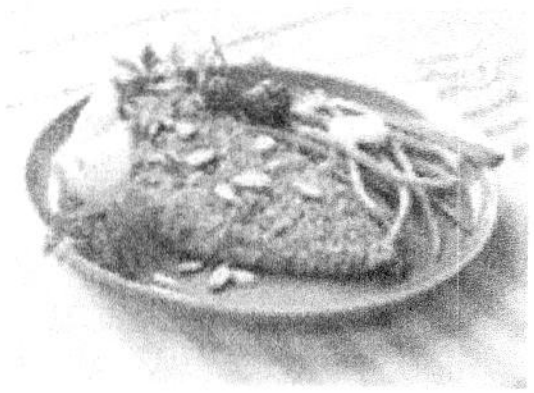

Cooking Instructions:

Preheat oven to 425°. Combine eggs and milk in a bowl and beat until fully blended. On a large flat plate, spread out breading mix, covering entire plate. Dip sole fillets one at a time in the egg mixture and place firmly on the Crispy Chicken Mix, covering fish completely on both sides. Repeat step with all fillets. Lightly grease a 3 qt baking dish with canola oil. Place sole in dish. Add sliced almonds to top of fillets. Dot each fillet with 1 Tbsp of Olivio or butter substitute without disturbing crumb and almond covering. Bake uncovered at 425° for 20 – 25 minutes or until golden brown.

Serve with green salad and grilled vegetables.

Serves 6 people.

Baked Ziti

Ingredients:

1 1/4 12 oz bags of Tinkyada Brown Rice Ziti Pasta Noodles
1 10 oz jar of gluten free pasta sauce
2 C shredded mozzarella cheese
1 lb ground sirloin, optional

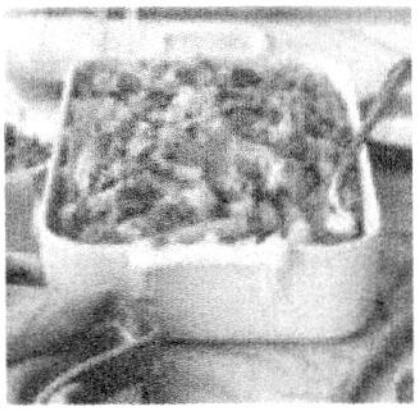

Cooking Instructions:

Boil pasta until tender. Do not overcook. Drain water, rinse with cold water and return to pot. Add 1 C of pasta sauce to pasta, mix and set aside. If adding meat, sauté meat in 2 Tbsp of olive oil or canola oil, drain, cool and mix into pasta evenly. In a 2 qt pan, add to the bottom a thin layer of pasta sauce. Cover then with a flat layer of pasta, top with a few spoonfuls of sauce and scatter a handful of mozzarella over it. Repeat step three times. Use the remainder of sauce over the top of pasta and top with a thicker layer of mozzarella. Bake at 350° for 45 minutes or until bubbling and topping is lightly browned.

Serve with green salad and gluten free garlic bread.

Serves 4 to 6 people.

Cheese Pizza

Ingredients:

1 16 oz package Bob's Red Mill Gluten Free Pizza Crust Mix
1 8 oz package shredded mozzarella cheese
1 1/2 C organic tomato sauce

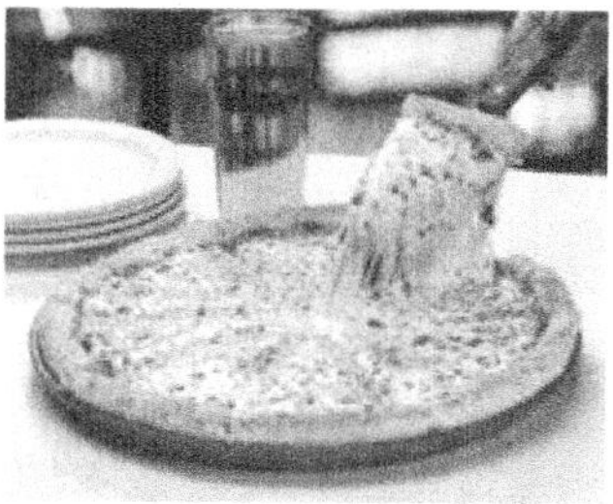

Cooking Instructions:

Preheat oven to 350°. Follow directions on the pizza crust package by mixing ingredients and letting it rise for one hour. Press dough onto a greased round 12 inch pizza pan, being sure to create a thicker crust at the edge of the pan. Bake at 350° about 15-20 minutes until lightly cooked. Remove from oven and let cool. Spoon in tomato sauce and spread onto the pizza shell until evenly covered, leaving just the thicker crust at the edge of the shell uncovered. Take a full handful of the shredded mozzarella cheese and shake it evenly onto the pizza shell. Repeat until it is evenly covered. For a lighter calorie pizza, use low fat cheese. Add whatever gluten free, nitrate fee meats or toppings you desire and bake at 350° for 25 – 30 minutes or until cheese and toppings are slightly golden brown. For a golden brown upper crust, paint with melted butter before baking.

Serves 4 people.

Chicken, Beef or Shrimp Stir Fry

Ingredients:

1 lb boneless, skinless chicken breasts (can also use sliced stir-fry beef or medium-sized cooked shrimp)
1 1/2 C cooked broccoli florets
1 1/2 C sliced, cooked baby carrots
1 C cooked pea pods
1/2 C water chestnuts
1/2 C chopped onion (optional)
1/3 C extra virgin olive oil
3/4 C Mr. Spice Ginger Gluten Free Stir Fry Sauce
1 Tbsp minced garlic (optional)

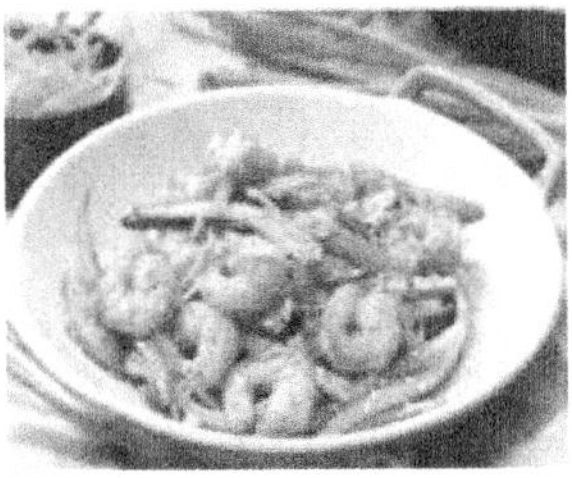

Cooking Instructions:

Cut each chicken breast into 5 strips and then again in half. Add the olive oil to a wok or a large frying pan. When oil is hot, add cut chicken and onions and sauté until cooked and lightly brown. Add cooked vegetables and water chestnuts and stir for 3 to 5 minutes, until mixture is hot. Add Stir Fry Sauce and garlic. Stir until fully mixed in and remove from heat.

Serve over brown rice, cooked gluten free noodles, or a bed of lettuce greens.

Chicken Divan

Ingredients:

6 boneless, skinless chicken breasts
1 C mayonnaise (can substitute Spectrum Canola Mayonnaise)
2 C "Full Flavor Foods" Vegetarian Mushroom Cream Soup
1 tsp sea salt
1/4 tsp gluten free garlic salt
4 C medium sized raw broccoli crowns
4 Tbsp white wine
1 1/2 C gluten free breadcrumbs

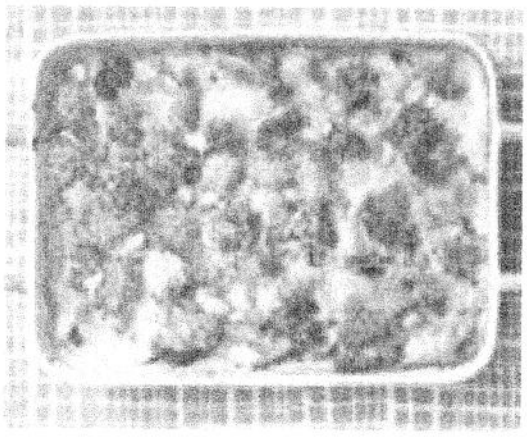

Cooking Instructions:

Preheat oven to 350°. Follow directions to make Mushroom Soup and cool. Combine mayonnaise, soup, sea salt, wine and garlic salt in a bowl and mix well. In a 30 oz glass baking pan, cover with a thin layer of the creamy mixture on the bottom and sides. Lay the raw broccoli crowns on the bottom of the pan until the pan is covered. Take tablespoons of creamy sauce and blob evenly over broccoli, saving 3/4 of mixture. Gently lay chicken breasts over broccoli. Cover chicken with the remainder of the cream sauce. Take handfuls of the breadcrumbs and shake them evenly to cover the entire top. Bake uncovered at 350° for 1 hour. Using a fork, stab the broccoli to make sure it has completely cooked.

Serves 6 people.

Chicken Parmigian

Ingredients:

6 boneless, skinless chicken breasts
1 1/2 10 oz jars of gluten free pasta sauce
1 12 oz container of gluten free bread crumbs
2 C shredded mozzarella cheese
6 oz shredded parmigian cheese
2 eggs

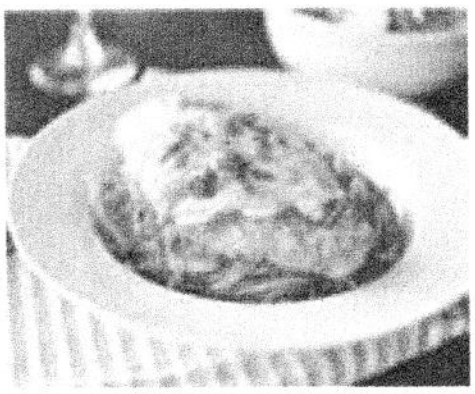

Cooking Instructions:

Preheat oven to 350°. Beat 2 eggs in a bowl and set aside. Combine parmigian cheese and bread crumbs, then spread them out on a large plate. Take each individual raw chicken breast and dip into the egg and cover both sides completely with bread crumb mixture. In a 30 oz glass baking pan, apply a thin layer of tomato sauce to bottom. Gently lay breaded chicken breasts into pan and cover with approximately 1 1/2 C of sauce. Shake mozzarella cheese evenly on top of the chicken and sauce. Bake covered for 45 minutes at 350°. Check and uncover and continue baking for 15 more minutes until bubbling and top is slightly browned.

Serve over gluten free pasta, with a salad and gluten free garlic bread or gluten free bread sticks.

Serves 6 people.

Chicken Pot Pie

Ingredients:

1 1/2 boneless, skinless raw chicken breasts
1 Perfect Pie Crust Mix from Gluten Free Pantry
2/3 C sliced cooked carrots
3/4 C diced cooked celery
1/2 C fresh peas
1 peeled and diced russet potato,
lightly boiled and cooled
2 1/2 C organic GF chicken broth
3/4 C Bob's Red Mill GF
All Purpose Baking Flour
1 tsp GF bouillon (optional for taste)

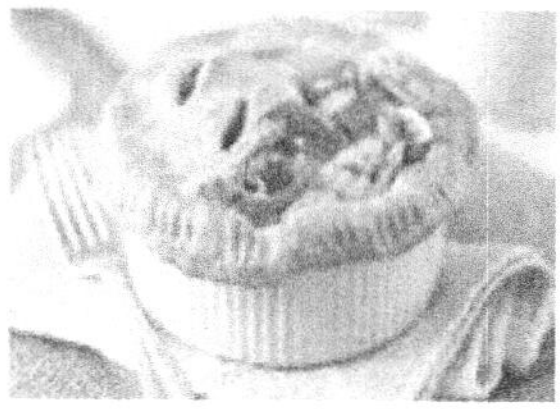

Cooking Instructions:

Preheat oven to 350°. Follow directions for the double crust pie, using two 8" pie pans, and set aside. Heat chicken broth until bubbles form. Reduce heat and slowly add enough flour and stir until mixture thickens into a gravy. Remove gravy mixture and set aside. Cut chicken breasts into 1/2" cubes. Combine carrots, celery, peas, potatoes, and chicken in a bowl and add gravy mixture. With a large spoon, toss the vegetables in the gravy until evenly distributed. Pour mixture into the pie shell evenly until mixture reaches just below the rim of the pie pan. Carefully remove second pie shell from pie pan and gently cover the mixture. With a fork, press gently around the edges of pie crust. Make four small slits in the top. Bake pie at 350° for 45 minutes or until golden brown.

Serves 5-6 people.

Chili

Ingredients:

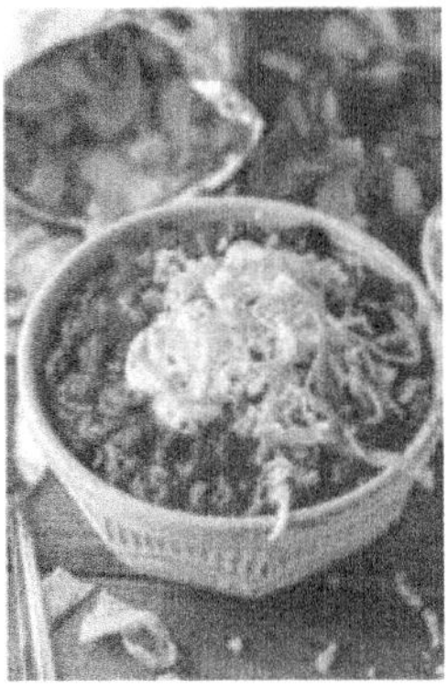

1 lb ground sirloin
1 large chopped yellow onion
28 oz can crushed tomatoes, drained
16 oz can of tomato sauce
2 16 oz cans of chili or kidney beans
2 Tbsp Bob's Red Mill Gluten Free Chili Powder

Cooking Instructions:

Sauté ground sirloin until brown and fully cooked, remove fat from pan and set aside. Chop and sauté onion until tender. Combine cooked onion, drained tomatoes, tomato sauce, drained beans, and chili powder and mix together. Add 3 Tbsp of water and cover. Cook on low to medium heat for one hour, stirring periodically. Add Gluten Free Masa Flour as a thickener if desired. Add 1 Tbsp of granulated cane sugar for optional sweetness. Garnish bowls of chili with chopped scallion, chopped onion, or shredded cheese.

Can be served with warmed Gluten Free Corn Bread.

Serves 6 people.

Crispy Chicken Strips

Ingredients:

1 lb boneless, skinless chicken breasts
1 1/2 C Kinnikinnick Crispy Chicken Mix (Gluten Free)
1 C fat free milk
1 egg
1/2 C extra virgin olive oil

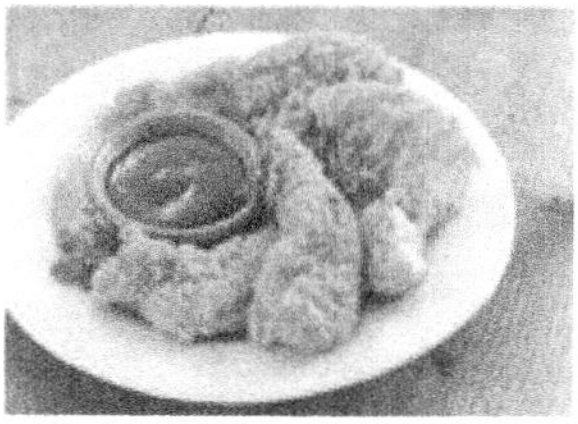

Cooking Instructions:

Heat oil in a frying pan at medium heat. Combine the milk and egg in a bowl and beat for 1 minute. Cut defrosted chicken breasts into 4 strips each. Dip chicken strips in the milk/egg mixture and then roll the strips in the Crispy Chicken Coating Mix. Place in the frying pan and cook until golden brown. Remove strips and drain excess oil.

Serve with potatoes, brown rice, over GF noodles or on bed of leafy lettuce or enjoy as a high protein snack.

Makes 2 servings.

Deep Dish Lasagna

Ingredients:

2 packages of Gluten Free Lasagna Noodles by Joy
16 oz fat free ricotta cheese
1 1/2 8 oz packages fat free or low fat
shredded mozzarella cheese
1 1/2 26 oz jars Classico Organic Tomato
Herbs and Spices Pasta Sauce
1/2 tsp sea salt

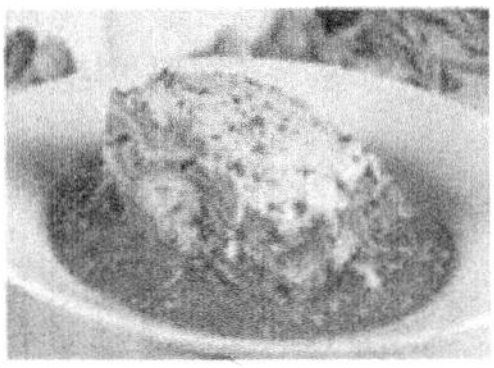

Cooking Instructions:

Preheat oven to 350°. Fill a large pot 3/4 full with cold water and heat on high to a full boil. Add sea salt and gently add lasagna noodles one by one to the boiling water. (Vary position of noodles to avoid sticking). After noodles are cooked, remove from heat and pour out water, quickly rinse with cold water, and set aside. Cover the bottom of a 9 x 12 x 3 inch pan with tomato sauce. Take approximately 3 full cooked lasagna noodles and place lengthwise, fitting closely to each other. Fill in any gaps with noodles so that the whole bottom is covered. On top of the noodles, add 1 inch blobs of ricotta cheese along the length of each noodle, approximately 4 blobs per noodle. Now sprinkle a handful of mozzarella cheese on top of the layer, sprinkling it evenly over the whole area. Dot with tablespoons of tomato sauce evenly over the cheeses. Add 3 more cooked lasagna noodles and repeat the same steps until the food is near to the top. Make sure the final top layer is solely pasta. Now paint with a thick layer of tomato sauce and top with 1 1/2 handfuls of shredded mozzarella. Cover with tinfoil and bake at 350° for 45 minutes. Remove tinfoil and bake for 15 more minutes until lasagna is bubbling hot and cheese is melted and slightly browned.

Serve with Gluten Free Italian or Garlic Bread or Breadsticks and a salad.

Serves 6 – 8 people.

Manicotti

Ingredients:

1 8 oz box of Tinkyada Brown Rice Grand Shells
1 C low fat ricotta cheese
1 C shredded mozzarella cheese
1/2 C parmesan cheese
1/2 tsp sea salt
1/4 tsp ground pepper
10 oz jar of tomato or
pasta sauce (gluten free)
2 tsp minced garlic

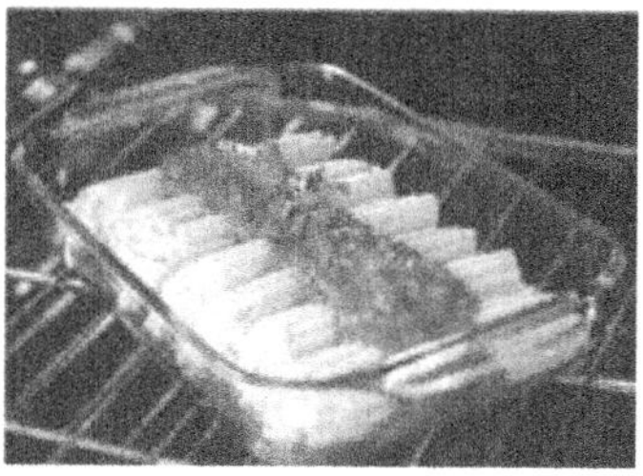

Cooking Instructions:

Boil 12 manicotti shells (more if your shells are small) until tender. Remove from water, rinse with cold water, drain and set aside. Preheat oven to 350°. Combine cheeses, sea salt, pepper, and garlic and mix well in a bowl. Gently spoon mixture into cooked shells. Arrange in a 3 qt (preferably glass) baking pan. Choose appropriate pan for however many shells you want to make. Spread a thin layer of tomato sauce onto bottom of pan. Place stuffed shells into pan evenly in rows. Spoon remainder of sauce over the top of shells. For a cheesier manicotti, add a handful of shredded mozzarella over the top of the shells and sauce. Bake at 350° for 25 – 30 minutes or until bubbling hot.

Serve with green salad and warmed gluten free Italian bread.

Serves 8 people.

Meatloaf

Ingredients:

1 lb ground beef
1 egg yolk or equivalent egg substitute
1/2 C chopped fresh parsley
1/2 C gluten free bread crumbs
1 tsp pineapple juice
1 tsp sea salt
1/2 C chopped onions
1/4 tsp ground pepper
1 1/2 Tbsp butter or substitute
3/4 C pine nuts
2 Tbsp gluten free catsup
1/2 C gluten free beef or vegetable stock

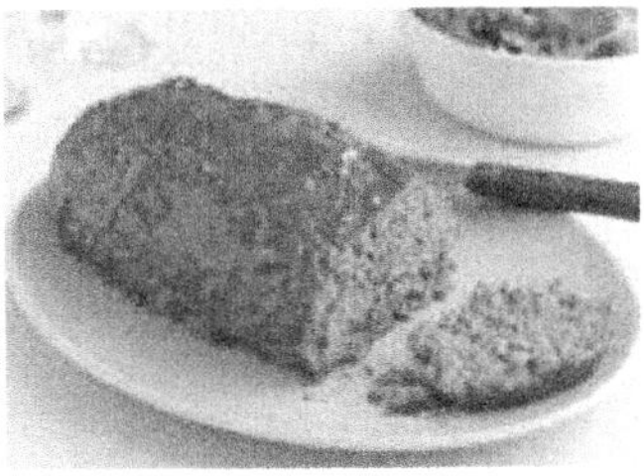

Cooking Instructions:

Preheat oven at 350° . Combine ground beef, egg yolk, breadcrumbs, pineapple juice, sea salt, pepper, onions, parsley, butter and pine nuts and knead evenly into a loaf shape and set aside. In a 9 x 5 x 3 inch nonstick or lightly greased pan, paint a transparent layer of catsup to bottom and sides. Press meatloaf slowly and evenly into the pan with the middle being slightly higher than the sides. Paint the top of the meatloaf with the remainder of the catsup. Sprinkle dried parsley on top. Bake uncovered at 350° for 1 hour. While baking, baste with 1/2 C gluten free beef or vegetable stock periodically. When meatloaf is done (crusty on the edges and cooked in the middle), pour excess fluid out of the pan and add all purpose gluten free flour to desired thickness for a gravy. You can add cooked sliced mushrooms to the gravy or pineapple juice for a hint of sweetness. Pour gravy over individual slices of meatloaf.

Serve with broccoli and carrots.

Serves 6 to 8 people.

Oriental Rice Wraps

Ingredients:

4 boneless, skinless chicken breasts
1 12 oz package Banh Trang Spring Roll Skins
1 1/2 C brown sugar (substitute brown rice syrup)
3/4 C fresh lemon juice
3/4 head iceberg lettuce
1 1/2 cucumbers
4 thinly sliced carrots
2 Tbsp minced garlic (adjust to taste)
2 Tbsp olive or canola oil

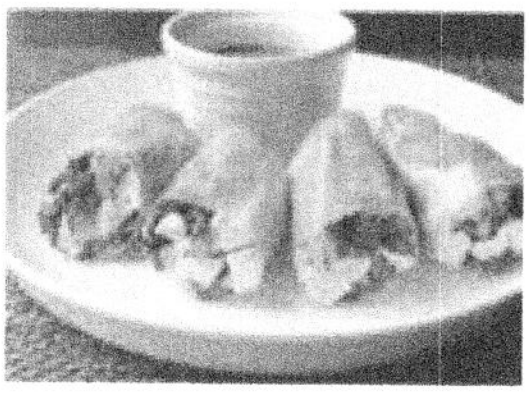

Cooking Instructions:

Slice chicken lengthwise into 1/4 inch slices and set aside. In a large, nonstick frying pan, sauté garlic with 2 Tbsp olive or canola oil. Add brown sugar and lemon juice. Add chicken and cook thoroughly. Cut lettuce into thin strips. Peel cucumbers, cut in half and slice lengthwise into very thin stalks. Remove 12 spring roll skins and run one at a time under warm water until soft, then place on large plate. (Keep separate so they don't stick.) Place lettuce and then carrots, cucumber and chicken with a teaspoon of the pan sauce into the center of a skin. Wrap ends over the stuffing first and then roll up the sides. Apply water to fuse the skin completely shut. Place in the form of flower petals on a large round serving platter. In the center of the platter, place a bowl of gluten free soy sauce, teriyaki sauce or sweet and sour sauce. Remainder of pan sauce can also be used for dipping.

Garnish dish with fresh small orchids.

Serves 6 to 8 people.

Potato Pancakes

Ingredients:

8 large russet potatoes
3 Tbsp raw, grated onion
3 eggs or equivalent of egg substitute
3 Tbsp Bob's Red Mill Gluten Free All Purpose Flour
1/2 tsp Hain Gluten Free Baking Powder
1 tsp sea salt
3/4 C olive or canola oil

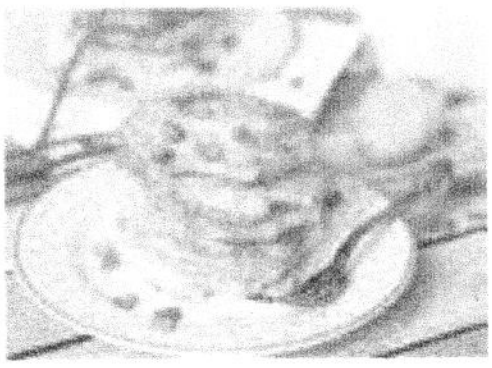

:

Cooking Instructions

Grate potatoes to measure 2 1/2 C. Remove excess fluid. Beat eggs and add to potatoes. Combine flour, salt and baking powder and mix evenly. Add flour mixture to potatoes and mix gently for 1 1/2 minutes until fully saturated. Add onion and mix again. In a large pan, add 3/4 C olive or canola oil and bring to a near boil. Drop Tbsp of potato mixture and brown on both sides, keeping centers slightly soft, but fully cooked. Remove from pan and drain excess grease onto paper.

Serve with organic apple sauce and garnish plate with parsley.

Serves 6 to 8 people.

Shrimp Tempura

Ingredients:

1 lb raw large shrimp
2 eggs or 3/4 C egg whites or substitute
3/4 C Bob's Red Mill Gluten Free All Purpose Baking Flour
3/4 tsp salt
1/4 tsp ground pepper
1 Tbsp olive oil or canola oil, plus
more to deep fry
1 tsp Braggs Amino Liquid Seasoning

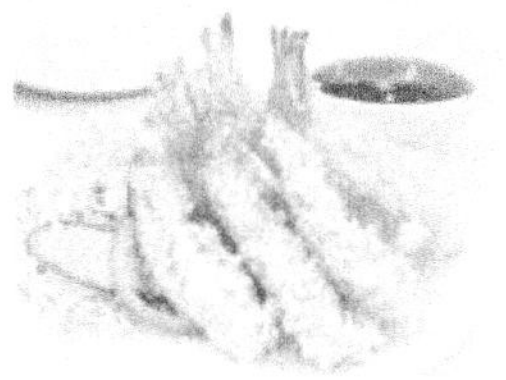

Cooking Instructions:

Shell, clean, and devein shrimp and remove the tails. Beat the eggs or egg product for 1 minute. Add flour, salt, pepper, oil, and Braggs Aminos to the egg mixture. Beat until all ingredients are combined and smooth. Immerse the shrimp one at a time into the mixture. Deep fry in olive or canola oil, heated to the point of small bubbles, until they are light brown. For thicker, crispier shrimp, repeat the dipping and deep frying a second time. Remove from oil and drain. Absorb residual oil on paper.

Serve with gluten free dressing, soy sauce, or lemon on a bed of fresh lettuce greens or rice noodles.

Serves 3 people.

Southwest Chicken

Ingredients:

6 boneless, skinless chicken breasts
1 12 oz bag of gluten free corn tortilla chips
2 15.5 oz jars chunky or fresh gluten free salsa
2 8 oz bags shredded cheddar or three cheese blend

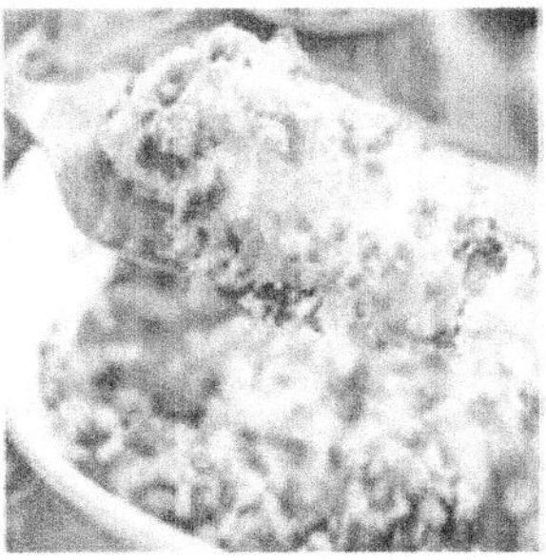

Cooking Instructions:

Cover bottom of a 30 oz glass baking pan with 3 Tbsp salsa. Add to pan one layer of whole tortilla corn chips. Shake two handfuls of shredded cheese over chips. Place chicken breasts in pan and cover with remainder of salsa. With two more handfuls of shredded cheese, cover chicken and salsa evenly. Bake uncovered at 350° for 1 hour.

Serve with green salad.

Serves 6 people.

Stuffed Cabbage with Brown Rice

Ingredients:

1/2 lb ground sirloin
1/2 head of green cabbage, uncut and boiled
4 Tbsp Braggs Aminos Seasoning Liquid
1 C cooked brown rice
4 Tbsp minced onions
3 Tbsp olive or canola oil
1/4 tsp sea salt
1/4 tsp paprika
1/4 tsp Gluten Free Curry Powder
1 C Mr. Spice Sweet and Sour Sauce

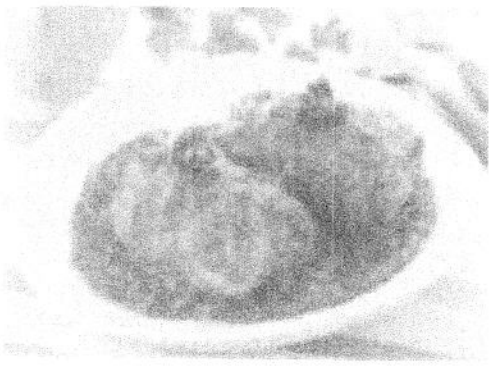

Cooking Instructions:

Preheat oven to 350°. Boil 8 large uncut cabbage leaves until tender and set aside. Sauté ground beef until fully cooked and browned. Add the brown rice, minced onions, sea salt, paprika, curry powder and Braggs Aminos Liquid. Fill each cabbage leaf with meat mixture and roll into a tight cylinder, tucking in the ends. Place in a baking pan and drizzle Gluten Free Sweet and Sour Sauce with some chopped onions and a hint of tomato sauce mixed in as desired for taste. Cover and bake at 350° for 40 minutes or until hot.

Add grilled vegetables if desired.

Serves 4 people.

Stuffed Pork Chops

Ingredients:

6 boneless, medium sized pork chops
1 package Barkat Sage and Onion Gluten Free Stuffing Mix
1 red apple
1 Tbsp gluten free garlic salt
1 tsp sea salt

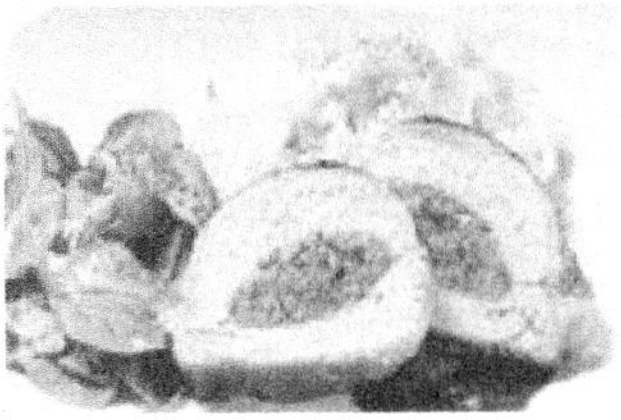

Cooking Instructions:

Preheat oven to 350°. Trim excess fat off the pork chops and cut a side pocket on each chop. Follow directions for the stuffing. Remove the skin and core of the apple and dice into 1/4 inch pieces. Mix salt and garlic salt and apple evenly through the stuffing. Insert 1/2 C of stuffing into each pork chop. Rub chops with olive oil and a pinch of salt and garlic salt. Place in lightly greased baking pan and bake uncovered at 350° for 45 minutes or until cooked through and lightly browned on top.

Serve with steamed vegetables.

Serves 6 people.

Tuna Noodle Casserole

Ingredients:

1 package of "Full Flavor Foods" Vegetarian Mushroom Soup Mix
1 1/2 6 oz cans of white tuna in water, drained
1 C of gluten free mayonnaise, if desired
2 7 oz bags of Cornito Gluten Free Egg Noodles
1/2 tsp sea salt
2 C crushed Gluten Free Cornflakes

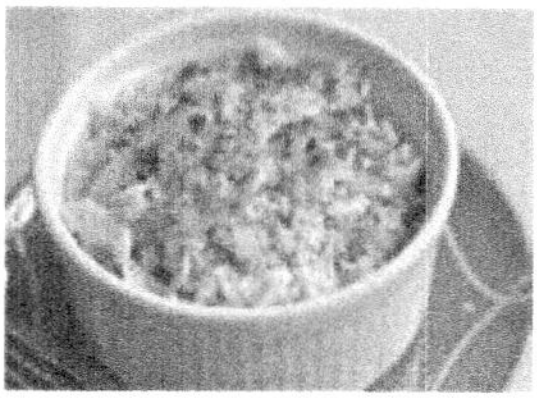

Cooking Instructions:

Preheat oven to 350°. Follow directions on soup and prepare to a thick, creamy consistency then let cool. Add mayonnaise and blend evenly. Add sea salt to mixture and blend thoroughly. Break apart tuna with a fork into small pieces and add to mixture. Set mixture aside in a large bowl. Boil both bags of noodles until tender, drain, and let cool. Gently fold noodles into tuna mixture and blend evenly. Fill 8 x 8 x 2 inch baking pan almost to the top. Put 2 C of Gluten Free Cornflakes in a plastic bag and crush into small pieces. Cover top of casserole completely with crushed cornflakes. Bake at 350° for 1 hour or until bubbling hot.

Serve with a green salad.

Serves 6 people.

Veal Marsala

Ingredients:

6 veal cutlets
4 Knorr Gluten Free Beef Bouillon cubes
2 C Bob's Red Mill Gluten Free All Purpose Flour
1 stick of butter (substitute 8 Tbsp butter alternative)
3 well beaten eggs
2 C boiling water
4 Tbsp Marsala wine
2 8oz bags Glutano Tagliatellle
Flat Noodles pinch sea salt

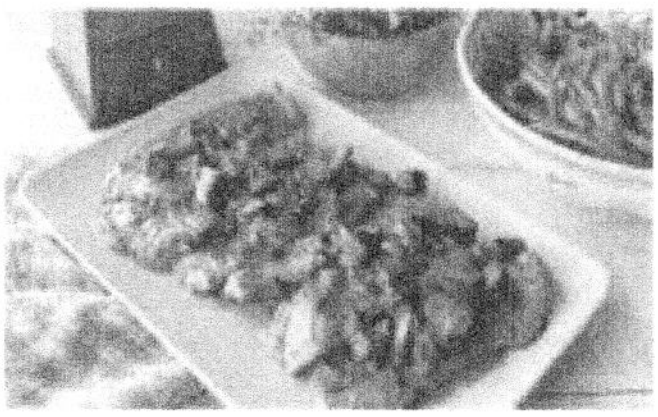

Cooking Instructions:

Bring large pan of water to a boil, add a pinch of sea salt and cook noodles until tender. Drain excess water set aside in a bowl covered to keep warm. Pound veal cutlets evenly without tearing the meat to about 1/2 inch thickness each and set aside. Dissolve 3 – 4 bouillon cubs in 2 C hot water and set aside. On a large plate, spread out flour evenly, covering the whole plate. Dip each cutlet into the beaten eggs and then place them one at a time in the flour, covering both sides thoroughly. In a nonstick large frying pan, melt butter over medium heat and place cutlets in pan, turning after lightly browned on each side. Do not overcook. After cutlets are cooked, cover them and set aside in a warm oven, but do not drain pan. Add to pan bouillon and wine and simmer over low heat, using small amounts of flour to lightly thicken sauce. Add sliced cooked mushrooms if desired. Remove veal from oven and place over a bed of noodles and cover with sauce.

Serve with steamed broccoli.

Serves 6 people.

A Gluten Free Resource For Meal Planning

My Favorite Gluten Free Sweets and Desserts

Funky Monkey Snacks
www.funkymonkeysnacks.com
(800) 783-1326
Freeze dried fruit snacks. Is a great alternative to chips and pretzels. Can be thrown into a homemade gluten free trail mix.

Gluten Free Brown Cow Yogurt
www.browncowfarm.com
(888) 429-5459
Certified gluten free yogurt except for the "Fruit and Whole Grains Product."

Sweet Sin Bakery
www.glutenfreedesserts.com
(410) 366-5777
Gluten free bakery and gourmet desserts.

Mototo Premium Desserts
www.mototodairyfree.com
+61 7 3391 0003
Dairy style desserts that are dairy, gluten, and soy free. An ice cream alternative.

"Natural Desserts" Vegan Jel Dessert
www.veganessentials.com
(866) 88-VEGAN or (252) 574-7761
Alternative to Jello.

Curious Cookie Gourmet
www.curiouscookie.com
(877) YUMMY-2-U (986-6928) or (973) 616-8500
Has a line of gluten free/lactose free/casein free gourmet cookies.

Foods by George Gluten Free Desserts
www.foodsbygeorge.com

NOTE: Some companies also have products containing gluten. These product lists are not limited to the categories stated.

(201) 823-0227
Frozen GF products usually found in the frozen sections of health food stores. Has a nice variety of muffins and desserts.

Gluten Free Bakery
www.glutenfreebakery.net
+61 7 3888 3289
Has extensive link to find a variety of desserts and baked goods, candy, and baking equipment.

Gluten Free Spice Network

Canadiagua Spice Co.
www.candaiguaspice.com
(585) 394-7840
Expanded to include a line of gluten free spices and also has GF cooking classes. Also has GF ready made meals.

Great American Spice Co.
www.americanspice.com
(877) 677-4239
Extensive list of Baking mixes and also has a variety of cooking oils to be used instead of extracts.

LBC Spice Co.
www.Luckyblackcatspiceco.com
(802) 763-2480
Seasonings, rubs, and spice blends.

Alchemy Spice Company
www.alchemyspiceco.com
(423) 322-2534 or (423) 322-0807
Cooking oils, mixes and spices.

Peacock Spice Company
www.peacockspices.com
(245) 565-1165
Spices from India and South East Asia.

The Relish In Spice Company
www.therelishinspicecompany.com
+44 20 1903 71076
Chutneys, sauces, puddings, and marinades.

The Spokane Spice Company
www.spokanespice.com
(509) 624-1490

NOTE: Some companies also have products containing gluten. These product lists are not limited to the categories stated.

Rubs and marinades, meat seasonings and cures. Has Gluten Free Bakery Equipment.

Uh Huh One Spice Blend Gluten Free
www.yankeegrocery.com
(203) 776-2091
All natural spice blend. Good alternative to salt.

NOTE: Some companies also have products containing gluten. These product lists are not limited to the categories stated.

Gluten Free Condiments

Annie's Naturals
www.Anniesnaturals.com
(800) 434-1234
Natural Salad Dressings, marinades, oils and vinegars, and condiments (must do a search for the Gluten free products).

Braggs Dressings and Seasonings
www.bragg.com
(800) 446-1990
All purpose seasoning and oils. All products are Gluten Free. Liquid Aminos are a good alternative to salt.

Mr. Spice
www.mrspice.com
(800) SAUCE-IT (728-2348)
Organic salt free sauces.

Orphee GF Mustards
www.maisonorphee.com
(800) 667-1530
Mustards and specialty oils and vinegars.

Premier Japan
www.edwardandsons.com
(805) 684-8500
Hoisin and Teryaki sauces.

San J
www.san-j.com
(804) 226-8333 or (800) 446-5500
Two organic Tamari wheat free soy sauces. One is low sodium.

NOTE: Some companies also have products containing gluten. These product lists are not limited to the categories stated.

The Really Great Food Company
www.reallygreatfood.com
(800) 593-5377
Gluten free, wheat free, soy free, dairy free, baking mixes (has extensive list of GF Products).

NOTE: Some companies also have products containing gluten. These product lists are not limited to the categories stated.

Breads and Mixes

The Birkett Mills
www.thebirkettmills.com
(315) 536-3311

Chebe Bread Mix
www.chebe.com
(800) 217-9510

Cybros, Inc.
www.cybrosinc.com
(262) 547-1821

GNF Foods
www.greatnorthfoods.com
(989) 356-2281 or (800) 968-0117

Gluten Free Mixes
www.glutenfreemixes.com
(866) 225-3432 or (503) 443-3803

Kirkman Foods
www.kirkmanlabs.com
(800) 245-8282 or (503) 694-1600

1,2,3 Gluten Free
www.123glutenfree.com
(843) 768-7231

Food For Life
www.foodforlife.com
(800) 797-5090 or (951) 279-5090

NOTE: Some companies also have products containing gluten. These product lists are not limited to the categories stated.

Flours

Authentic Foods
www.authenticfoods.com
(310) 366-7612

Bob's Red Mill
www.bobsredmill.com
(800) 349-2173

Gifts of Nature
www.giftsofnature.net
(888) 275-0003

Special Foods
www.specialfoods.com
(703) 644-0991

Dowd and Rogers
www.dowdandrogers.com
(916) 451-6840

Arrowhead Mills
www.arrowheadmills.com
(800) 434-4246

NOTE: Some companies also have products containing gluten. These product lists are not limited to the categories stated.

English Muffins, Dinner Rolls, Buns, Tortilla Wraps

Foods By George
www.foodsbygeorge.com
(201) 612-9700

Gillians Foods
www.gilliansfoods.com
(781) 586-0086

Glutafin
www.glutafin.co.uk
0800 988 2470

Quejos Cheesebuns
www.quejos.com
(604) 420-0832

Cybros Small Sandwich Buns
www.cybrosinc.com
(262) 547-1821

Food For Life
www.foodforlife.com
(800) 797-5090

NOTE: Some companies also have products containing gluten. These product lists are not limited to the categories stated.

Cereals, Waffles, Granola

Alti Plano Gold
www.altiplanogold.com
(415) 380-5050

Amazing Grains
www.simplyamazinggrains.com
(303) 428-4421

Dietary Specialties
www.dietspec.com
(888) 640-2800

Gluten Free 4 Me
www.glutenFree4me.com
(717) 899-5120

Liprofin
www.shs-nutrition.com
+44 15 1228 8161

Perky's Natural Foods
www.perkysnaturalfoods.com
(888) 4-PERKYS (737597)

Van's All Natural
www.vansintl.com
(323) 585-5581

Bakery On Main Rainforest GF Granola
www.allergygrocery.com
(800) 891-0083

NOTE: Some companies also have products containing gluten. These product lists are not limited to the categories stated.

Gluten Free Goji Berry Granola
www.reallygreatfoods.com
(800) 593-5377

Lifestream Wildberry GF Waffles
www.naturespath.com
(604) 940-0505

Bagels, Breadsticks, Baguettes, Hamburger/Hotdog Rolls

Against The Grain
www.againstthegrainslc.com
(801) 955-4418

Gluten Free Bagel Co.
www.glutenfreebagelcompany.com
(888) 458-8360

Enjoy Life Foods
www.enjoylifefoods.com
(888) 50-ENJOY (36569)

Glutino
www.glutino.com
(800) 363-3438

Outside The Breadbox
www.outsidethebreadbox.com
(719) 633-3434

Allergy Grocery
www.allergygrocery.com
(800) 891-0083

Elo Peto
www.elpeto.com
(800) 387-4064 or (519) 650-4614

NOTE: Some companies also have products containing gluten. These product lists are not limited to the categories stated.

Breadcrumbs, Coverings and Coatings

Dakota Lakes Products
www.dakotalakes.com
(701) 952-2611

Fortitude Gluten Free
www.fortitudeglutenfree.com
(866) NO-GLUTEN

Kinnickinnick
www.kinnickinnick.com
(877) 503-4466

Natural Food Works
www.naturalfoodworks.com
(530) 756-1862

Gillians Foods
www.gilliansfoods.com
(781) 586-0086

Holgrain
www.holgrain.com
(800) 551-3245

Orgran
www.orgran.com
+61 3 9776 9004

NOTE: Some companies also have products containing gluten. These product lists are not limited to the categories stated.

Crackers and Biscuits

Blue Diamond Growers
www.bluediamond.com
(916) 442-0771

Edward and Sons
www.edwardandsons.com
(805) 684-8500

Mary's Gone Crackers
www.marysgonecrackers.com
(530) 846-5100

Glutino
www.glutino.com
(800) 363-3438

Gluten Free Life
www.Glutenfreelife.com
(300) 794-170

Kame
www.kame.com

NOTE: Some companies also have products containing gluten. These product lists are not limited to the categories stated.

Dip, Dip Mixes, Batters

Dippy Chick
www.dippychick.com
(603) 686-5536

Yankee Grocery
www.yankeegrocery.com
(203) 776-2091

Delightfully Delectable
www.delightfullydelectable.com

New England Cupboard
www.newenglandcupboard.com
(207) 941-1152

Gina's Gourmet Creations
www.ginasgourmetcreations.com

Prairie Moon Soup Mixes
www.pmsoup.com
(866) 331-0767

Frontier Soup Mixes
www.frontiersoups.com
(866) 300-SOUP (7687)

NOTE: Some companies also have products containing gluten. These product lists are not limited to the categories stated.

Pastas

Adrienne's Products
www.adriennesgourmetfoods.com
(805) 964-6848

Glutafin
www.glutafin.co.uk
0800 988 2470

Mayacamas Fine Foods
www.mayacamasfinefoods.com
(707) 291-3024

Mrs. Leepers
www.mrsleepers.com
(973) 338-0300

Rizopia
www.rizopia.com
(416) 609-8820

Tinkyada Brand
www.tinkyada.com
(416) 609-0016

Olive Nation
www.olivenation.com
(781) 989-2033

NOTE: Some companies also have products containing gluten. These product lists are not limited to the categories stated.

Pizzas, Pizza Crusts, Mixes

Madwoman Foods
www.madomanfoods.com
(612) 825-6680

Dad's Gluten Free Pizza
www.glutenfreepizza.com
(208) 922-3005

Azna Gluten Free Pizza Crusts
www.aznaglutenfree.com
(530) 677-5810

Toovaloo Gluten Free
www.toovalooglutenfree.com
(800) 291-8386

Pizza Pizza
www.pizzapizza.com

Bob's Red Mill
www.bobsredmill.com
(800) 553-2258

Arrowhead Mills
www.arrowheadmills.com
(800) 434-4246

Vertoris
www.vertorispizza.com
(941) 751-0333

Still Riding Pizza
www.stillridingpizza.com
(203) 683-7238

NOTE: Some companies also have products containing gluten. These product lists are not limited to the categories stated.

Matteo's Pizza
www.matteospizza.com
(615) 661-5811

Glutino Frozen Pizzas
www.glutino.com
(800) 363-3438

Pie Crusts, Mixes

Natural Feast
www.naturalfeast.com
(866) 628-6346

Breads From Anna
www.breadsfromanna.com
(319) 354-3886

Gluten Free Pantry
www.glutenfree.com
(800) 291-8386

Arrowhead Mills Graham Pie Crust
www.arrowheadmills.com
(800) 434-4246

NOTE: Some companies also have products containing gluten. These product lists are not limited to the categories stated.

Snacks, Nutrition, Energy Bars

Alpsnack
www.alpsnack.com
(877) 786-3649 or (760) 743-2211

Bumble Bar
www.bumblebar.com
(509) 924-2080

Gluten Free 4 Me
www.glutenfree4me.com
(717) 899-5120

Jat Foods
www.jatfoods.com
(805) 322-5192

Liprofin
www.shsnutrition
+44 15 1228 8161

Omega Smart
www.omegasmartbar.com
(603) 425-6800

Sunflour Baking Co.
www.sunflourbaking.com
(916) 488-4150 or (888) 610-3708

Can Do Kid Gluten Free Kids Snacks
www.iamacandokid.com
(888) 207-0567

Kind Energy Bars
www.kindsnacks.com
(212) 616-3006

NOTE: Some companies also have products containing gluten. These product lists are not limited to the categories stated.

Perfect 10 Bar
www.perfect10bar.com
(604) 540-1000

Snacks, Nutrition, Energy Bars cont.

Grabem Snacks
www.grabemsnacks.com
(732) 469-8833

Arico Foods
www.aricofoods.com
(866) 98-ARICO

Really Great Foods
www.reallygreatfoods.com
(800) 593-5377

Mr. Spice Popcorn
www.mrspice.com
(800) 728-2348

Pure Fit
www.purefit.com
(866) PURE-FIT

NOTE: Some companies also have products containing gluten. These product lists are not limited to the categories stated.

Canned Soup, Soup Mixes, Broths, Soup Bases

Frontier Soups
www.frontiersoups.com
(800) 300-7687

Scandinavian Spice Co.
www.scandinavianspice.com
(877) 783-7626

Wellness Grocer
www.wellnessgrocer.com
(888) 272-8775

Amy's Kitchen
www.amyskitchen.com
(707) 568-4500

Better Than Bouillon
www.superiortouch.com
(909) 923-4733

Prarie Moon Soup
www.pmsoup.com
(866) 331-0767

Shelton's
www.sheltons.com
(909) 623-4361

NOTE: Some companies also have products containing gluten. These product lists are not limited to the categories stated.

Beverages

Bard's Tale Beer
www.bardsbeer.com
(877) 440-2337

Cloud County Tea Company
www.cloudcountyteas.com
(785) 446-3639

The Ramapo Valley Brewery
www.ramapovalleybrewery.com
(866) 932-5918

Iateapie Cinnamon Hot Chocolate and Smoothies
www.iateapie.net

Bernard Foods
www.bernardfoods.com
(800) 323-3663

NOTE: Some companies also have products containing gluten. These product lists are not limited to the categories stated.

Frozen Meals

Cuisine Solutions
www.cuisinesolutions.com
(703) 270-2900

Everybody Eats Inc.
www.everybodyeatsinc.com
(718) 369-7444

Glutino
www.glutino.com
(800) 363-3438

Quality Frozen Foods Inc.
www.qualityyfrozenfoods.com
(718) 256-9100

Amy's Kitchen
www.amys.com
(707) 568-4500

Ian's Natural Foods
www.iansnaturalfoods.com
(800) 54-FOODS (36637)

NOTE: Some companies also have products containing gluten. These product lists are not limited to the categories stated.

Shelf Stable Meals

Hormel
www.hormelfoods.com
(800) 523-4635

Tasty Bite
www.tastybite.com
(888) 827-8900

Go Picnic
www.gopicnic.com
(777) 328-2490

Allergaroo
www.allergaroo.com
(314) 604-2210

AAOOB Storable Foods
www.aaoobfoods.com
(888) 201-6785

Orgran
www.orgran.com
+61 3 9776 9004

Minsley Inc
www.minsley.com
(909) 458-1100

Lundberg Family Farms
www.lundberg.com
(530) 882-4551

NOTE: Some companies also have products containing gluten. These product lists are not limited to the categories stated.

Made in the USA
Monee, IL
16 September 2025

25816555R00030